CANCER FIGHTING FOODS:

Everything You Need To Know About The Main Effects And Properties Of Food In The Fight Against Cancer

DONG LA

ISBN: 9781658868716

Legal & Disclaimer

inside this book. You agree that by continuing to read this book, where appropriate and/or necessary, you shall consult a professional (including but not limited to your doctor, attorney, or financial advisor or such other advisor as needed) before using any of the suggested remedies, techniques, or information in this book.

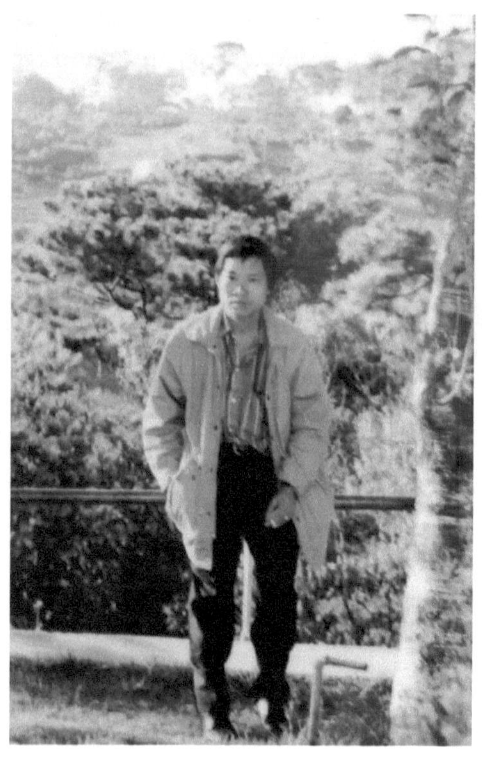

-DONG LA -

(Writer and Pharmaceutical Chemical Researcher)

TABLE OF CONTENT

INTRODUCTION

Although the science is constantly evolving, new cures have been invented, many new medical devices have been made, and many new drugs have been produced, the number of people who get sick and die from cancer is still constantly increasing in the world.

According to WHO (World Health Organization), the number of deaths due to cancer ranks second globally and in 2018 there were about 9.6 million deaths. The cost of curing cancer is very expensive and rising. In 2010, the total cost of cancer treatment in the world was estimated at approximately US$ 1.16 trillion.

About one-third of cancer deaths are due to leading behavioral and dietary risks including eating fewer vegetables and fruits. (Source: https://www.who.int/news-room/fact-sheets/detail/cancer)

Why does everyone know that consuming food is closely linked to cancer risk but that people still don't eat properly? Is it because people have not understood the scientific nature of the problem that food has properties that can prevent and fight cancer? If people understand those valuable healing properties of food, they will be motivated and positive for choosing the right food for meals.

To suffice this need for knowledge, this book presents the scientific bases of using food at meals to prevent and fight cancer.

From the onset and progression of cancer tumors, researchers have identified the causes and conditions for their development and also found the weapons that can fight this dangerous disease.

If we imagine that treating cancer is like a battle with different attack directions, then interestingly, fruits, vegetables, and medicinal plants can participate in all of those directions.

The attack directions are:

1. Against mutagenesis that causes cancer

Food and supplements can fight the genetic mutation of DNA caused by agents such as radiation, toxic chemicals and oxidants (free radicals) of metabolic processes in the body.

2. Anti-angiogenesis of cancer tumor

Cancer cells are created by the genetic change of normal cells, do not go through apoptosis (programmed cell death), divide uncontrollably, and grow very quickly into tumors. Therefore, the tumor creates many new blood vessels that provide nutrients to nourish it. The idea of preventing blood vessel proliferation so that the tumor is not nourished, starving it, is the basis of a new treatment, a therapeutic revolution, called Anti - angiogenesis. Anti-angiogenic drugs are called targeted drugs. Researchers also discovered that many fruits, vegetables, and medicinal plants also have anti-angiogenic properties, and tested them to treat cancer.

In this book, there is a story of a woman, Kathy Mydlach Bero, who defeated breast cancer with anti-angiogenic diet.

3. Neutralize the acidic environment of the cell that causes cancer

This book also presents controversial issues about the debate for nearly a century about the invention of Otto Warburg. Otto Heinrich Warburg, who was awarded the 1931 Nobel Prize, discovered that cancer was due to "the replacement of oxygen respiration in normal body cells by fermenting sugar."

After nearly 80 years of controversy and debate, several researchers from the United States have had research results supporting the Warburg's theory.

Some tests, which identify tumors on PET scans, have used radioactive glucose and found that cancer cells attract glucose faster than non-cancer cells. This process suggests cutting off sugar supply can starve and kill cancer cells. Researchers have proposed a diet that minimizes the number of carbohydrates and sugars, and they are replaced by good fats such as olive oil and other vegetable oils. Because fats that go through digestion do not produce sugar that nourishes cancer, but still generate energy for normal cells to function.

According to Warburg, the lack of oxygen provided to cells causes anaerobic respiration which is the fermentation process that produces lactic acid. Lactic acid causes an acidic cell environment to turn normal cells into cancer. Thus the cell's acidic environment acts in some way as a mutant that alters the genetic characteristics that have caused the abnormal proliferation of cancer cells. From that scientific basis, researchers also found that regular and adequate use of fruits and vegetables at meals can also prevent and treat cancer because they can neutralize the acidic environment of the cell.

The research result of scientists today not only validates the Warburg's theory but also lift the mystical veil of Eastern medicine.

"Circulating "qi" and blood" is a treatment principle of oriental medicine that has existed since ancient times. Eastern medicine concept that when the "*qi*" and blood circulate of course the body will not pain, on the contrary, when the "*qi*" and blood do not circulate of course the body will pain. "*Qi*" here is the term for both oxygen and energy. Practicing Yoga and Qi gong brings many health and spiritual benefits to the practitioner, and if we understand the scientific nature of the practice, we will know that breathing and exercising properly can also be a way to prevent and fight cancer. And as such, the air is the most valuable medicine and no payment to buy.

4. Reverting the epigenetic changes causing cancer

Epigenetics are phenotypic changes that can be inherited without being involved in a change in the DNA sequence. Abnormal epigenetic changes also cause many types of cancer. These abnormal epigenetic changes can be reversed with "*epigenetic drugs.*" These drugs are also found in the nutrients and biological substances of the food we eat.

***

Those are the main attack directions on the anti-cancer front. Fortunately, the Creator generously provided us with many weapons to use in that battle.

The author also boldly mentions opposing views and discusses with those who have them, such as critique ideas about Warburg theory regarding the use of alkaline foods to prevent cancer.

Dietary cancer prevention and treatment may be a practical solution because not everyone can afford expensive cancer treatment. Everyone can practice a healthy diet based on local crops. We can make our own decisions to do what doctors can't do for us. It is the use of food so that food is not only nutritional but also chemotherapy.

However, we must understand that no one food is a miracle drug that can prevent and cure cancer. Moreover, although it is easy to buy foods, it is difficult for us to follow a healthy diet regularly because of our lifestyle and taste. Therefore, we must be very determined to be successful in using regular diets with just enough amount of meat and plenty of vegetables, tubers, and fruits, the best way for our body to be healthy and prevent cancer. We choose foods and how to cook them so that every meal is not only a party to enjoy the smell, taste of the delicious dishes but also a preventive and curative one.

February 12, 2020

DONG LA

CHAPTER I: THE FOODS ARE RESISTANT TO MUTATIONS THAT CAUSE CANCER

1. Mutation Cause Cancer

Mutations are the most common cause of genetic changes that alter the nucleotide sequence of DNA that causes cancer. Mutagens include high-energy electromagnetic radiation, chemicals, and oxidizing agents, and alkylating agents.

A series of mutations in the genes of DNA can cause cancer. The researchers identified and classified genes into two broad categories: oncogene and tumor suppressor.

A carcinogenic gene is a mutated gene and when they are active at high levels, it will cause cancer.

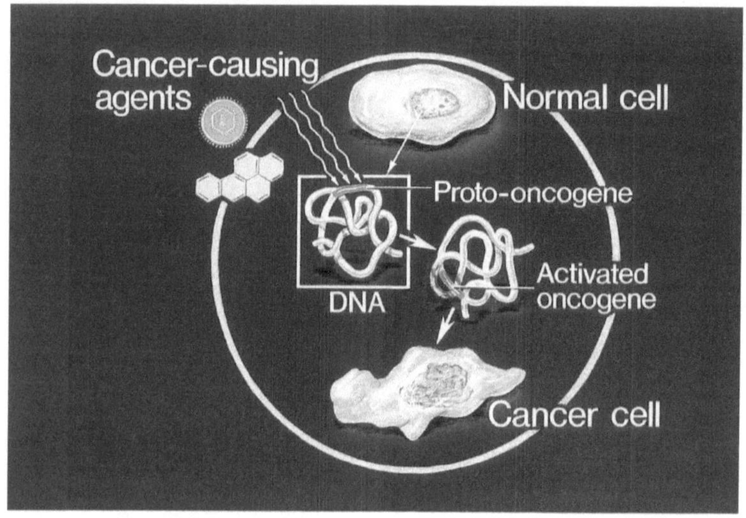

(Source: https://en.wikipedia.org/wiki/Oncogene)

Tumor suppressor genes are those that inhibit cell division, repair DNA errors or notify cells through apoptosis (programmed cell death). When tumor suppressor genes are mutated, malfunctioned, the cells will grow out of control, possibly forming cancerous tumors.

2. The Foods and supplements against the mutation of radiations

One of the first known mutants is radiation. Artificial radiation sources (in nuclear reactors) or natural radioactive elements (such as radon and uranium) can also damage DNA or other cellular components.

DNA can be broken down by X-rays and lead to different types of chromosomal damage. Ultraviolet radiation (UV) can cause point mutations.

Foods and supplements that can help protect the body and resist the effects of radiation. Our body's susceptibility to radiation and Diet are closely intertwined. Radiation and pollutants damage vitamins, calcium, essential fatty acids, etc. If our meals provide enough of these substances, they will become a barrier that protects our bodies from the negative effects of radiation and pollutants. Therefore, there is a list of foods and supplements that help balance our body chemistry.

Chlorophyll, a green substance, is readily available because it is found in most green leaves, including the green vegetables we eat every day. Barley grass, chlorella, and other vegetables are rich in chlorophyll and other supplements such as essential fatty acids, proteins (amino acids), enzymes, and vitamins. Chlorophyll is a key component in the process of photosynthesis, which sustains plant life and produces oxygen for the atmosphere, has a big role to play in the health of the Earth.

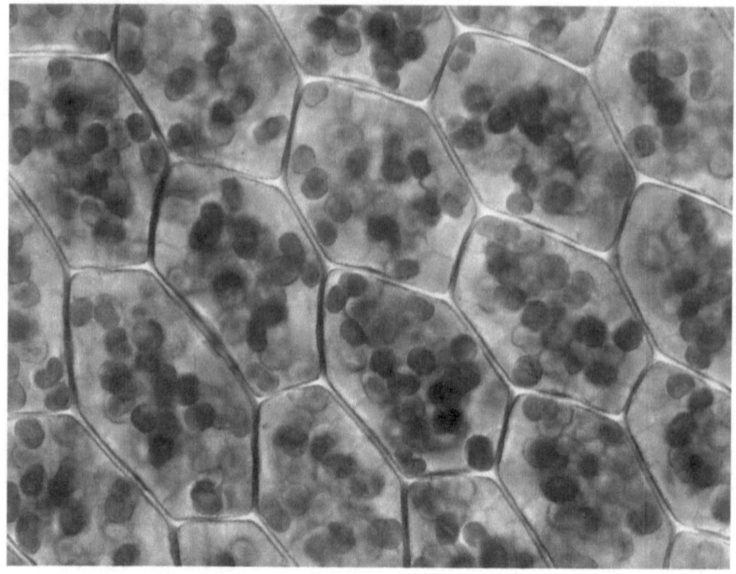

(Source: https://www.nationalgeographic.org/encyclopedia/chlorophyll/)

Many studies have shown that chlorophyll can inhibit radiation, can protect animals from harm when they are irradiated. In addition, chlorophyll can detoxify the liver and other organs of the body, support wound healing, etc.

Miso made primarily from naturally fermented soybeans. It is the whole source of protein that provides the body, promotes health and helps neutralize radiation pollution. The Japanese, who were exposed to radiation after two atomic bombings in Hiroshima and Nagasaki, ate miso daily and did not have cancer.

Sea vegetables can make agar that can be used to protect the human body from radioactive effects.

The supplements used to protect the body include Vitamin A or beta carotene; Vitamin C + bioflavonoids & rutin; Vitamin E; Coenzyme Q10; Proanthocyanidins (Grape seed extract/Pycnogenol; DHEA; Melatonin; Calcium/ magnesium; Zinc; Selenium; etc.

3. The effect of nutrition against chemical mutations

Various chemicals can also cause mutations. They bind to DNA and interfere with the replication or transcription. For example, benzo-a-pyrene in tobacco smoke and aflatoxin are often found in moldy agricultural products.

Chronic inflammation produces mutagenic chemicals that can lead to DNA damage, such as hepatitis virus infection.

Many diseases, including cancer, are caused by unfavorable genetic mutations that damage DNA. In the majority of them are not inherited. They appear only due to exposure to environmental agents. Luckily, researchers have proved a range of natural compounds in fruits, vegetables and medicinal plants that can prevent damage by mutations to protect the DNA.

3.1. Chlorophyll, Flavonoids, Carotenoids

a. Chlorophyll

Among the natural compounds, chlorophyll, in addition to anti-radioactive mutant properties, is also one of the most promising agents that can protect DNA against deadly gene mutations due to mutant chemicals.

Chlorophyll has been used as a medicine to treat diseases, including cancer. It is insoluble in water, so people semi-synthesized from chlorophyll into chlorophyllin that has a stronger effect. The remarkable anti-cancer effect of chlorophyllin is its dose to prevent cancer much lower than other natural compounds. If people take Chlorophyllin daily, it will be an excellent protection substance against a variety of compounds that can cause cancer. People have produced products from chlorophyll and sold them on the market.

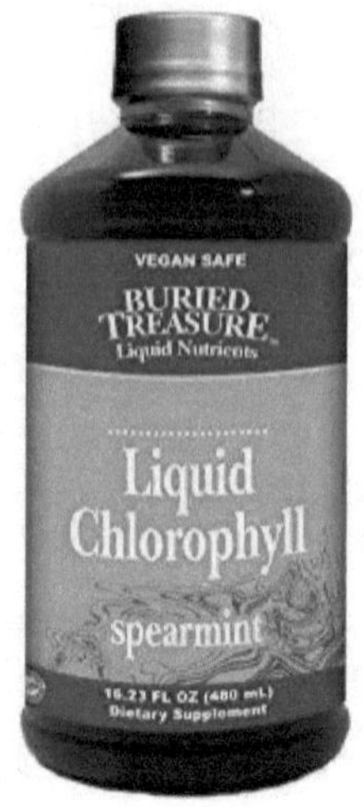

(https://www.google.com/search?q=Chlorophyll&source)

When we cook food, we create a variety of DNA attackers including benzopyrene. Well-done meats—fried, grilled, or barbecued chicken, pork, and beef with skin—contain the powerful carcinogens 2-amino-1-methyl-6-phenylimidazo [4,5-b] pyridine and benzopyrene.

Chlorophyllin can counter the carcinogenic effect of benzopyrene as follows:

It limits the reaction to produce benzopyrene-DNA adducts - molecular formed when DNA is attacked by a carcinogen, degrades the carcinogen formed when benzopyrene is metabolized by the body, reduces the activity of enzymes in the liver that convert benzopyrene to carcinogens and stimulates enzymes to convert benzopyrene into harmless substances. Many studies have documented the capacity of chlorophyllin to prevent the mutagenic activity of carcinogens. Chlorophyllin may help prevent pancreatic, colon, breast and liver cancers. For leukopenia, chlorophyllin is more effective than vitamin C, and it has the same effect as leucogen without any side effects. And chlorophyllin may against the radiation harmful effects

Other compounds found in foods that also have anti-mutagenic effects include Vitamins (Vitamin C, Vitamin E, and Vitamin A) and a document written that:

"Several authors have suggested that natural antimutagens may belong to any of the following major class of compounds. Major emphasis has been laid on the flavonoids, phenolics, carotenoids, coumarins, anthraquinones, tannins, terpenoids, saponins and several others all of which are secondary plant metabolites. More than 500 compounds belonging to at least 25 chemical classes have been recognized as possessing antimutagenic/protective effects."

(Source: https://scialert.net/fulltextmobile/?doi=rjmp.2011.116.126)

b. Flavonoids

Flavonoids are polyphenolic molecules that are a group of plant metabolites found in many fruits and vegetables.

In addition to the various beneficial biological properties, they have a high ability for anti-mutation. Flavonoids of Citrus juice have antimutagenic and anti-cancer effects. The activity of other flavonoids (found in Psorothamnus fremontii, Millingtonia hortensis, Glycyrrhiza glabra, Ocimum javonica) has been tested against types of mutations.

Medicinal plants and natural foods contain many types of phenolic compounds. In raspberries, strawberries, walnuts, grapes, etc. whose ellagic acid is antimutagenic. Green tea and black tea also have epicatechin, (-) - epigallocatechins, (-) - epicatechin gallate, (-) - epigallocatechin gallate are compounds with anti-mutant activity. Curcumin in turmeric and eugenol in cloves can also inhibit the mutagenicity.

c. Carotenoids

Organic solvent extracts of several carotenoid-rich fruits and vegetables such as tomatoes, yellow-red peppers, carrots, brussels, and apricots were tested. They can inhibit some mutations caused by aflatoxin B1, benzo pyrene, etc.

Also, compounds such as Anthraquinones, Diterpenoids, Coumarins, Tannins, etc. have been tested to prove they can resist mutations.

We cannot avoid mutations due to environmental pollution, harmful substances in food and improper lifestyles. Mutations can cause serious illnesses that are difficult to treat, such as cancer. Therefore, it is important to resist mutations by using regular fruits and vegetables that have anti-mutagenic substances during meals.

4. The antioxidants in food

Oxidizing agents are a kind of mutagen. Oxidants such as hydrogen peroxide or free radicals make multiple forms of damage, particularly of DNA double-strand breaks. These breaks are the most dangerous because these are difficult to repair and can make point mutations, deletions from the DNA sequence, insertions, and chromosomal translocations. Therefore, they can cause cancer.

Free radicals are produced by many processes within our bodies. They are entities that have lost an electron, come from the breakdown of foods, from the breakdown of toxins and they enter our bloodstream. During normal aerobic metabolism also produce several reactive oxygen species (ROS), including hydrogen peroxide, superoxide and hydroxyl radical. Exposure of cells to radiation can also produce free radicals.

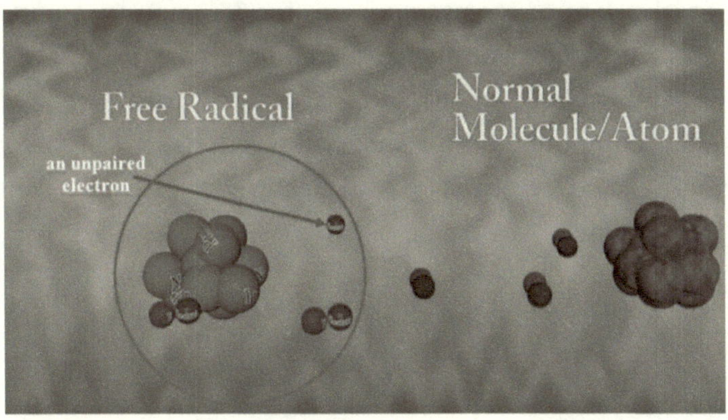

All ROS can able to interact with cellular ingredients containing DNA bases or the deoxyribosyl backbone of DNA to generate damaged bases or strand breaks. Radicallinked damage of proteins and DNA plays a major role in the development of aging and degenerative diseases such as arthritis, neurodegenerative disorders, arteriosclerosis, and cancer.

When these free radicals attach themselves to the lining cells of the arteries, they cause injury. The body trying to heal the injury, platelets will try to plug that injury and making a clot that can cause myocardial infarction or stroke.

Antioxidants, therefore, become very important because they are the electron donors for free radicals and can neutralize them.

Fruits and vegetables contain high levels of antioxidants. Phytochemicals are antioxidants and divide into different groups such as astaxanthin, lycopene's, xanthine, carotenoid pigments, carotenoids, and other phytochemicals.

There are also other substances act like functional foods such as polyunsaturated fatty acids-PUFAs and amino acids, probiotic, prebiotic and synbiotic. Their antioxidant value largely comes from polyphenolic and anthocyanoside and additionally they compose of other flavonoid antioxidants such as beta-carotene.

Some of the natural compounds in foods, especially antioxidant compounds in plants, can reduce the damage caused by free radicals to DNA that is believed to be the root cause of most cancers. Antioxidant compounds can reduce mutagenesis by both decreasing oxidant-stimulated cell division and decreasing oxidative damage to DNA.

4.1. Some antioxidants: Astaxanthin, Lycopene, Resveratrol, Lutein, Probiotic

a. Astaxanthin

Astaxanthin found in red foods such as salmon, crab, lobster, and crawfish, as well as in algae and krill oil, is a valuable antioxidant. It is a fat-soluble carotenoid pigment, gives certain marine animals and plants their pink or red colors. Astaxanthin does not only scavenge free radicals but also restricts the production of free radicals. Astaxanthin can offer protection against the effects of ultraviolet (UV) when people are exposed to sunlight. Astaxanthin is capable of providing nerve protection as it can cross the blood-brain barrier and scavenge free radicals in the brain.

Researchers have called Astaxanthin "the king of antioxidants" because of its antioxidant capacity, which is about 100 to 6,000 times more than other antioxidants such as Vitamin E, Vitamin C, beta-carotenoids, lutein, and zeaaxanthin. Therefore, studies are showing that astaxanthin is effective against inflammation and many types of cancer. For example, studies have shown that astaxanthin or lycopene can inhibit the increase of prostate cancer in humans. Astaxanthin has been produced in the form of pure supplements and sold on the drug market.

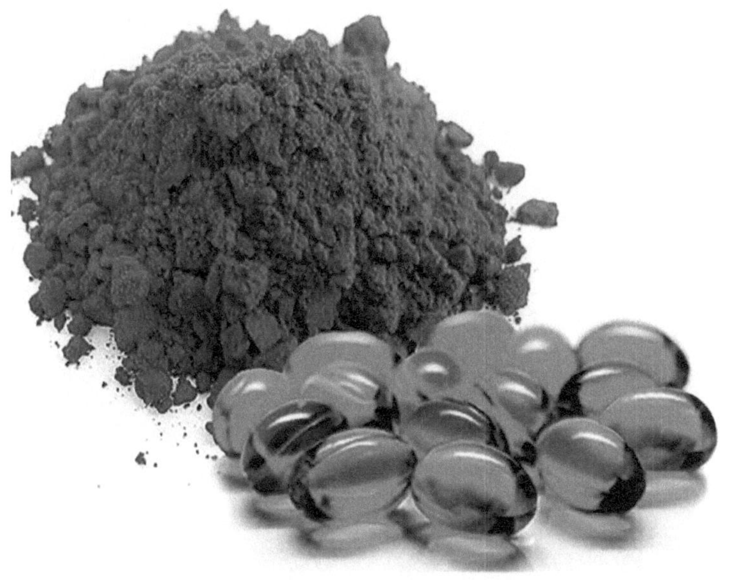

(Source: https://www.google.com/search?q=Astaxanthin)

b. Lycopene

Tomatoes have a characteristic red color of Lycopene which is contained in this fruit. Watermelon, apricot, grapefruit, pawpaw, pink guavas and tomatoes contain lycopene and people absorb lycopene mainly from tomatoes at meals. Lycopene can reduce the concentration of low-density lipoprotein and cholesterol.

Lycopene's single group oxygen neutralizing capacity is 10 times higher than alpha-tocopherol and with beta-carotene, twice as high. Researchers have demonstrated that people use lycopene-rich foods regularly have anti-inflammatory effects, against the risk of cardiovascular disease and cancer. Based on research results, lycopene prevents cancer cells from growing stronger than ß and α-carotene. The anti-cancer ability will increase if using a combination of ß-carotene and lycopene. Combining tomatoes containing lycopene with garlic containing S-allylcysteine will reduce the risk of stomach cancer. Lycopene has a special effect to prevent the increase of prostate cells with cancer.

It has also produced lycopene products and marketed them.

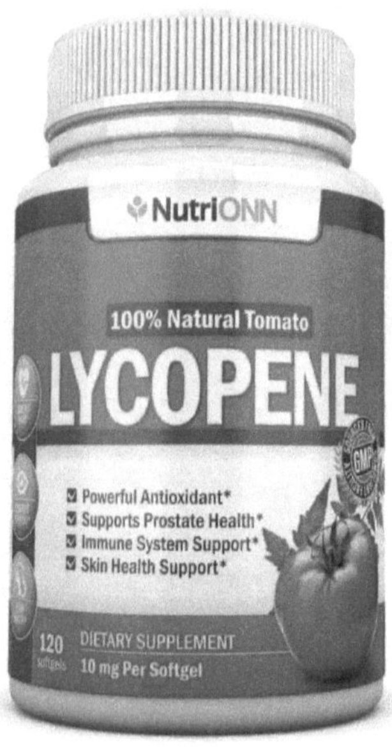

(Source: http://www.nutrionn.com/product/lycopene/)

c. Resveratrol

Red grapes and wine made from them contain resveratrol, a very powerful antioxidant. This powerful antioxidant has been praised by many nutritionists for its effectiveness in slowing down aging, decreasing the chances for heart disease and cancer. It also can eliminate free radicals, viruses, and bacteria, reduce the risk of cell destruction from radiation and repair DNA. We need to drink some red wine every day for good health.

d. Lutein

Lutein is very strong antioxidants in the eye lens, can oppose cell damage and the development of cancers by neutralizing free radicals. Lutein is abundant in green leafy vegetables such as spinach, different kinds of squash and zucchini (or vegetable marrow); colored vegetables such as sweet corn, sweet peppers, and peas; many fruits such as kiwi, grapes, and orange; and egg yolk. Lutein can reduce the risk of cancer, interacts with the mutagens 1-nitropyrene and aflatoxin B1.

***

In addition, all of the following substances have the ability of antioxidant, neutralization of free radicals, so they are all effective against cancer.

Carrots are the tubers that contain the most α-carotene, followed by pumpkins and winter squash; the β-carotene found in yellow fruits, orange, green leafy vegetables, and other vegetables; the β-cryptoxanthin has found in oranges, papayas, peaches, mangoes, nectarines, watermelon, grapefruit, plums, black olives, red bell peppers, and tangerines; canthaxanthin is found in several blue-green algae, green algae, annular seabream (Diplodus annularis), crustacea, golden mullet (Mugil auratus), carp (Cyprinus carpio), etc; Fucoxanthin is a naturally occurring orange-colored or brown pigment and found in diatoms (Bacillariophyta), brown seaweeds (Phaeophyceae); Isothiocyanates are the phytochemicals containing sulfur and found in cruciferous vegetables such as broccoli, kale, cauliflower, cabbage, Brussels sprouts, and others.

e. Probiotic

Probiotic are living microorganisms which have positive effects on human health because of the improvement of the balance of the intestinal microflora. Probiotics are also effective in preventing cancer because they inhibit intestinal Helicobacter pylori which generate carcinogenic substances.

***

There are randomized controlled clinical trials that do not give evidence that antioxidant supplements in the diet are beneficial in preventing primary cancer. (Cite: https://www.cancer.gov/about-cancer/causes-prevention/risk/diet/antioxidants-fact-sheet). Some researchers have explained that the effects of some antioxidants in the form of purified chemicals contradict their effects when they are used in food along with a mixture of vitamins and minerals. In some cases, oxidants are excreted too quickly after being ingested.

Therefore, the effects of antioxidants are synergistic and gradual, we must use foods with antioxidant active ingredients regularly and long-term to get good results.

CHAPTER II: THE MEDICAL REVOLUTION AGAINST ANGIOGENESIS OF CANCER TUMORS

1. What is Angiogenesis?

Angiogenesis is the process of creating new blood vessels from previously existing blood vessels. The blood vessels that circulate blood carry oxygen and nutrients that nourish billions of cells in the body.

A tumor starts from a cancer cell that divides rapidly in number. In the early stages, these cells use blood vessels near them. As the tumor grows, it invades nearby tissues, spreading to other organs in the body (metastatic process). The tumor needs more blood vessels to give it nutrition; without angiogenesis, it could only grow to one half a cubic millimeter in size.

If the cancer cells are not supplied with blood, they will only form microscopic cancer tumors. Autopsy studies of people who have died in car accidents show that there are microscopic cancer tumors in their bodies. Without a blood supply, most of these cancers tumors will never become dangerous. But once angiogenesis occurs cancers can grow exponentially. Cancer cells can circulate in blood vessels as metastases. In the late stages of cancer, when angiogenesis is turned on, the cancer cells will grow continuously like wild.

The idea of preventing blood vessel proliferation so that the tumor is not nourished, starving it, is the basis of a new treatment called Anti-angiogenesis.

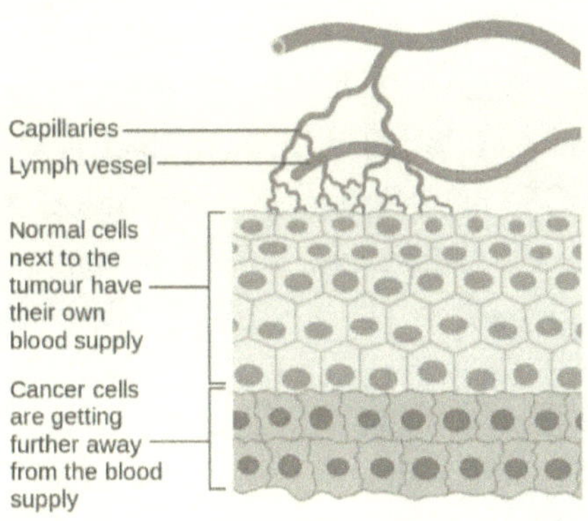

(Source:

https://en.wikipedia.org/wiki/Angiogenesis#/media/File:Diagram_showing_why_cancer_cells_need_their_own_blood_supply.svg)

Judah Folkman was the first to propose the concept of "antiangiogenesis" in 1971. He thought that the process of creating new blood vessels of the tumor in the early stages can be inhibited, leading to the ability to prevent tumor development and metastasis.

The proliferation of endothelial in normal blood vessels differs from that in tumor vessels. There are very few normal endothelial cells and very rarely they are duplicated compared to that of endothelial cells in the blood vessels of cancer tumors, so the rate of duplication of endothelial cells of the tumor blood vessels much faster than that of normal blood vessels. Therefore, agents that selectively resist angiogenesis which nourishes the tumor do not damage normal blood vessels.

Research to find ways to prevent angiogenesis that nourishes tumors has been considered a medical revolution in recent years.

Anti-angiogenic therapy is completely different from chemotherapy because it selectively targets the blood vessels that are nourishing cancer. Therapists can do this because the tumor's blood vessels are not the same as normal healthy blood vessels. They are very poorly constructed and therefore, they are very vulnerable to the treatments that target them. Cancer cells can secrete chemicals (such as angiogenin, vascular endothelial growth factor (VEGF), fibroblast growth factor (FGF) ...) stimulates new blood vessel generation. From that basis, researchers have studied to create drugs that hinder the process of angiogenesis. Those drugs called targeted drugs, such as bevacizumab, sunitinib, sorefenib...

Researchers always warn that our diet is one of the causes of cancer. So we need to change our diet, we could remove from our diet what to strip out take away. On the contrary, we can add to our diet what are naturally anti-angiogenics that can beat back the blood vessels that nourish cancer. So, like a paradox, we can eat food to starve the cancer cells making them die.

Researchers have found that hundreds of natural and synthetic substances have been identified as capable of antiangiogenesis.

Many fruits, vegetables, tubers, spices, seeds, and other foods contain substances that are biologically active, including anti-angiogenic. For example, Green tea contains epigallocatechin-3-gallate (EGCG); Soybeans contain genistein; grapes contain resveratrol; Tomatoes, papayas, and watermelon contain lycopene; sardines, anchovies, mackerel, herring, trout, and salmon contain omega-3 polyunsaturated fatty acids; Cruciferous vegetables such as kale, bok choy, brussel sprouts, radishes, mustard greens, collard greens, cauliflower, broccoli, and cabbage contain glucosinolates; Thyme, beets, parsley, onions, and spinach contain flavonoid; In fermented products such as natto (fermented soy), yogurt and cheese contain menaquinone (vitamin K2); Turmeric contains curcumin, a flavonoid; Papaya contains beta-cryptoxanthin; and etc.

2. Can we eat to starve cancer cells?

"William W. Li, MD, is a doctor, scientist, speaker, and author of "EAT TO BEAT DISEASE – The New Science of How Your Body Can Heal Itself". He is best known for leading the Angiogenesis Foundation. His TED Talk, "Can We Eat to Starve Cancer?" has garnered more than 11 million views."

(Source: https://drwilliamli.com/)

During that presentation, he said:

"We've discovered is that Mother Nature has created a large number of foods and beverages and herbs with naturally-occurring inhibitors of angiogenesis."

He showed the image in an experiment proving that an extract from red grapes containing the active ingredient resveratrol inhibited abnormal angiogenesis by 60% and said strawberries, soybeans, and there is a growing list of foods that are resistant to angiogenesis.

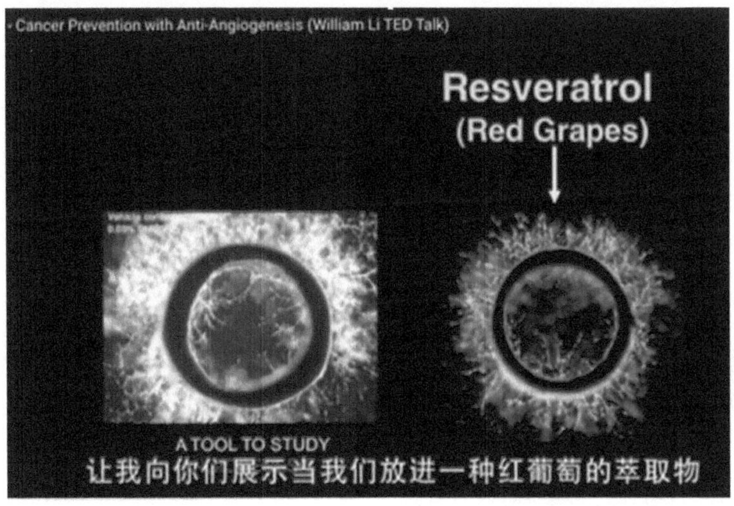

He also said that, in the laboratory, researchers compared the effectiveness of some anti-angiogenic drugs with foods; The results show that: "...in some cases, they're more potent than the actual drugs: soy, parsley, garlic, grapes, berries"; "A study of 79 thousand men followed over 20 years in which it was found that men who consumed cooked tomatoes two to three times a week at up to a 50% reduction in their risk of developing prostate cancer. Tomatoes are a good source of lycopene and lycopene is anti-angiogenic."

(Source: https://www.youtube.com/watch?v=kTDQb1MwzOo)

3. The story of a woman winning cancer with anti-angiogenic foods

There was a woman who told a very interesting, still new story (2018): she changed her diet, used anti-angiogenic foods, which helped her to win her fight against breast cancer.

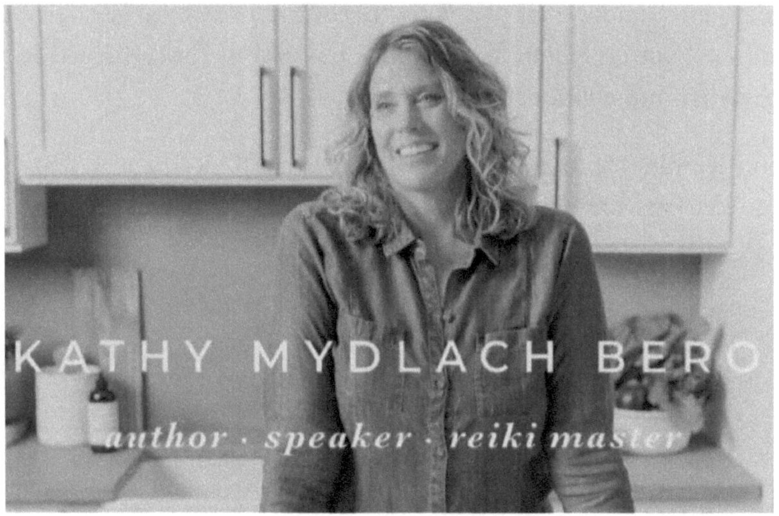

She is Kathy Mydlach Bero, a Wisconsin woman, is 41 years old and mother of two daughters. In 2005, Bero was diagnosed with breast cancer by doctors and only lived for about 21 more months.

She was treated with surgery, radiation, and chemotherapy. However, she did not recover. The drugs she had taken were ineffective.

At that time, a friend advised her to learn and use anti-angiogenic foods.

Anti-angiogen foods are foods that when people eat them, they can prevent cancer tumors from creating new blood vessels so that cancer can easily spread. Those foods are carrots, purple potatoes, leeks, walnuts, berries, green tea, and garlic, a spice, which is considered to be the most important anti-angiogenic drug.

"When a recipe calls for two cloves, I'm probably going to put in six because garlic is a really strong cancer fighter," Bero said.

(Source: https://www.wavy.com/news/national/using-food-as-medicine-womans-battle-against-cancer-being-studied-by-harvard-researchers/)

Today, after more than 12 years Bero has breast cancer, that diet combined with meditation and other training methods helped her to recover from the illness.

Upon learning of Bero's success, at Harvard University, researchers planned to research her special diet that could cure breast cancer.

CHAPTER III: THE ACID – BASE BALANCE OF THE AVIRONMENT AROUND CELLS AND CANCER

1. The debate for nearly a century about the invention of Otto Warburg, the cause of cancer

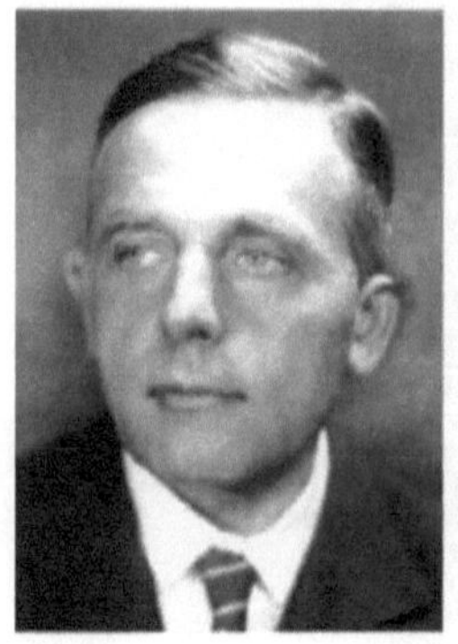

(Source: https://www.annandachaga.com/blogs/news/92184966-dr-otto-warburg-discovered-cause-of-cancer)

In 1931, Otto Heinrich Warburg was awarded the Nobel Prize for the invention of the cause of cancer. According to that invention, the main reason for cancer is that oxygen respiration of normal cells is replaced by sugar fermentation due to disturbed mitochondrial function.

In one of his lectures, he stated: *"... the prime cause of cancer is the replacement of the respiration of oxygen in normal body cells by a fermentation of sugar."*

(Source: http://healingtools.tripod.com/primecause1.html)

All cells of the body need energy to survive and function. With normal cells, the energy is supplied by oxygen respiration, aerobic metabolism of nutrients. According to Warburg, cancer cells, not like that, get energy by anaerobic respiration, which is the fermentation of glucose sugar, the product of food digestion.

He said numerous experiments have shown that food lacking respiratory enzymes will cause impairment of cellular respiration. If food is added to these enzymes, they will repair respiration.

He proposed a cure for the disease. Saturation of all body cells with oxygen is the first and foremost condition. The second important thing is to stay away from external carcinogens that cause loss of capillary circulation causing impaired cellular respiration. He claimed reality proved that when cell respiration was not impaired, cancer cells would not exist.

According to him, anaerobic metabolism that provides energy for cancer cells to survive and grow, so they only live in environments with low oxygen levels and cannot live at high oxygen levels. Therefore, it is necessary to increase blood circulation, need high hemoglobin concentration in the blood and always add respiratory enzymes to food, while eliminating exogenous factors that cause cancer, can prevent the types of cancer.

Warburg firmly claims that the main reason for cancer is due to the lack of oxygen of cellular respiration which creates the acidity around cells in the body. Hence he proposed that high acidity around the cell is united to not only cancer growth but also causes many other diseases such as osteoporosis, diabetes and heart disease.

However, unlike Warburg thought and to this day, the main reason for cancer is thought to be mutations in oncogene and tumor suppressor gene. The change in cell metabolism (the fermentation that creates the acidic environment of cells) is the result of cancer, not the cause that Warburg conceived.

When Warburg was frustrated because his idea lacked acceptance, he cited a sentence he thought was Max Planck's words: *"Science advances one funeral at a time."*

(Source: https://en.wikipedia.org/wiki/Otto_Heinrich_Warburg)

But after nearly 80 years of controversy and debate, researchers from Boston College at Washington Medical University reported their new findings in the study of mouse brain tumors (published in the Journal of Lipid Research) have supported Warburg's theory.

(Source: https://www.sciencedaily.com/releases/2009/01/090112093334.htm)

In his work, *The Metabolism of Tumours*, Warburg demonstrated that all forms of cancer are characterized by two basic conditions: acidosis and hypoxia (lack of oxygen), *"Lack of oxygen and acidosis are two sides of the same coin: where you have one, you have the other."*

(Source: https://sites.google.com/site/ganodermareview/the-root-cause-of-cancer)

From this scientific basis, people have come up with cancer treatments based on the principle of *"the body's acid-alkaline balance."*

The energy supplied to the body works through the metabolism of nutrients that occur in cells. The metabolic process produces ATP, energy-carrying molecules and cells can only use energy from ATP.

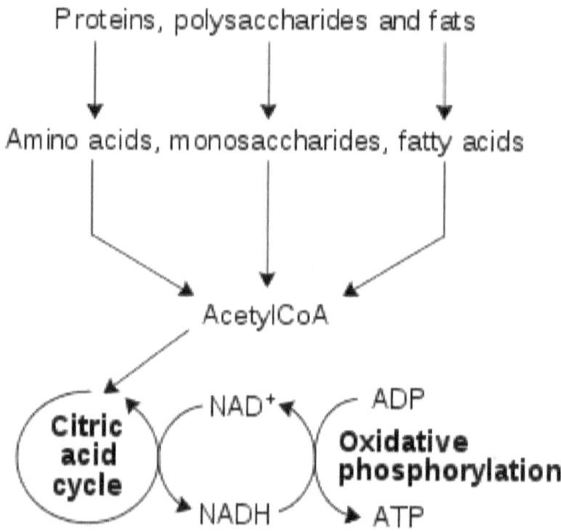

(Source: https://en.wikipedia.org/wiki/Metabolism)

In the body, ATP is synthesized by two different pathways: anaerobic and aerobic processes. With the normal activities of a healthy person, ATP is created mainly by the aerobic process, but when people are a vigorous and prolonged activity or the frail elderly are affected by weather or illness, etc. the respiration process does not provide enough oxygen for all cells, ATP is also generated by the anaerobic process. This anaerobic process also produces lactic acid, which increases the acidity of the environment where cells lack oxygen.

The human body has a slightly alkaline pH, in the range of 7.35 - 7.45. This is tightly regulated by the process of urinary excretion of the kidneys. Depending on what we eat, the pH of urine will change. However, that may not be possible due to poor kidney function because of various causes such as illness, aging or our diet. For example, when the patient's blood circulation is poor in a certain organ of the body, the respiration of the cells will lack oxygen, creating lactic acid. The lactic acid will cause pain if not excreted. It is this stagnated lactic acid that increases the acidity of the blood and cells, leading to further reductions in oxygen levels in cells, which according to Warburg are the cause of cancer.

To this day there are still many who oppose the Warburg hypothesis. They claim that cancer cells create acidic environments rather than acidic environments that create cancer cells:

"And while tumors grow faster in acidic environments, tumors create this acidity themselves. It is not the acidic environment that creates cancer cells, but cancer cells that create the acidic environment."

(Source: https://www.healthline.com/nutrition/the-alkaline-diet-myth)

Warburg's lecture *"The Prime Cause and Prevention of Cancer"* shows that the above view misunderstood Warburg's invention. In that lecture, he said he focused on answering the question of how normal cells of the body can turn into anaerobes.

He said that if the mouse cells were placed in culture medium with saturated oxygen pressure, in vitro, they would develop into pure aerobes without any sugar fermentation. Opposite, if the oxygen pressure is reduced to inhibit oxygen respiration, within 48 hours, the aerobic respiration of mouse embryonic cells during the division of the two cells would be changed into the fermentation of cancer cells.

(Source: http://healingtools.tripod.com/primecause1.html/)

The acidic environment is the environment of many hydrolysis reactions, so the increased acidity of the environment around the cells can cause hydrolysis reactions that change the structure of genes or chromosomes. Thus, the acidity of the environment around cells can be considered as a mutant agent such as radiation, chemicals, and free radicals.

Those who followed the Warburg hypothesis wrote that the cause of the illness due to acid-alkali imbalance is not a new concept.

In 1933, Dr. William Howard Hay of New York, in his innovative book, *The New Era of Health*, wrote that body acidosis caused all kinds of illnesses.

More recently, Dr. Theodore A. Baroody has said the same idea in his book, Alkalize or Die: *"A multitude of illnesses don't matter. The problem is they all come from the same cause ... too much tissue acid waste in the body!"*

(Source: https://ionizers.org/acidosis.php)

Very early in the mid-19th century, researchers discovered that rabbit urine was more acidic when fed primarily meat, and conversely, more alkaline when given Eat mostly plants. From that result, they claim that the pH of blood depends on the composition of waste products in the metabolism of cells. Similar to the burned things that leave ash, the metabolism of the nutrients from food in the cells also leaves "ash", metabolic waste. Some researchers think that acid ash is the causative agent, whereas alkaline ash is considered the protective agent. From this ash hypothesis, the researchers classified food.

2. The food classification by alkalinity and acidity for the purpose of cancer prevention

According to the ash hypothesis, food has been classified into two groups that are acidic or alkaline for healing purposes based on the acid-base balance in the blood.

Foods that are considered to be acidic include: meat, fish, eggs, dairy, grains, alcohol, etc.

 Foods that are considered alkaline include fruits, vegetables, nuts, legumes, etc.

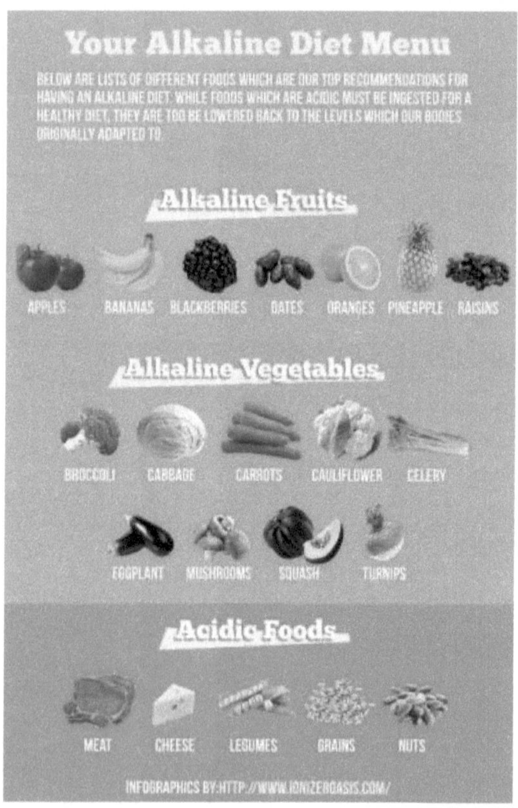

(Source: https://trendingposts.net/trending-health-news/amazingknow-why-an-alkaline-diet-may-cure-cancer/)

Our human body has billions of cells that are all slightly alkaline and must maintain this alkalinity to function normally and stay healthy.

However, cellular metabolism produces energy-carrying molecules, metabolic products and metabolic wastes, many of which are naturally occurring acids, such as lactic and uric. The buildup of these acids will cause illness and pain. Lactic acid will cause pain and uric acid will cause gout disease, and they create a bad acid environment for the body. The body must neutralize this high acidity before it can cause toxicity around and in the cell. If the amount of acid exceeds the body's ability to regulate, then alkaline foods will supplement the body to perform that neutralization process.

There are many opinions of organizations as well as individuals in the name of science who oppose the hypothesis that metabolic "ash" affects the pH of blood. They believe that food affects the pH of urine, not blood, because when the blood is excessively acidic or alkaline, the kidneys will immediately excrete them into the urine, or the opposite, absorb to neutralize. This function of the kidney is called acid-base homeostasis. If the pH is abnormal, people will die.

However, people with such views need to understand that homeostasis is only maintained in perfectly healthy people. When the metabolic waste is too much but the kidneys are weak, the acidity, not of the whole body but only in areas where cellular respiration is lack of oxygen, will be high. This increased acidity is not lethal enough; it only gradually causes degeneration in various organs, causing diseases including cancer.

They also need to understand that when people eat alkaline food and drink alkaline water not to increase the alkalinity of the blood in the whole body but to provide the alkaline substances that the body lacks to neutralize excess acid, stabilize standard pH. Indeed, foods cannot change the normal value of pH in blood; they only change their abnormal value.

Although people, who oppose both the Warburg hypothesis and the idea of using high blood pH neutralization with alkaline foods for disease prevention and treatment, they still wrote the following:

"As you can see, the myth of the need to make the body more alkaline does not have significant value with respect to cancer cell growth or development. However, we do know that incorporating more alkaline-type foods is recommended. The American Institute for Cancer Research recommends a plant-based diet which aims at receiving at least five servings of fruits and vegetables per day (at least 2 ½ cups), using whole grains versus refined grains, incorporating beans/legumes more often and meat less often. Incorporating these dietary habits will limit your intake of acidic foods, increase your intake of alkaline foods, and provide your body with the cancer-fighting nutrients it craves".

(Source: https://mnoncology.com/about-us/practice-news/acid-alkaline-balance-and-cancer-the-truth-behind-the-myth/)

***

Also from Warburg's invention: cancer cells survive and grow thanks to the energy of glucose fermentation, researchers have proposed a diet to treat cancer. It is a diet that minimizes the number of carbohydrates and sugars, and they are replaced by good fats such as olive oil and other vegetable oils. Because fats that go through digestion do not produce sugar that nourishes cancer, but still generate energy for normal cells to function.

3. Warburg theory and ancient oriental medicine

Experimental results by researchers from Boston College at Washington Medical University not only supported Warburg's theory but also lifted the mystery veil covering Eastern medicine.

"Circulating "qi" and blood" is a treatment principle of oriental medicine that has existed since ancient times. Eastern medicine concept that when the "*qi*" and blood circulate of course the body will not pain, on the contrary, when the "qi" and blood do not circulate of course the body will pain. "*Qi*" here is the term for both oxygen and energy. This is true according to modern science. When the circulating blood does not bring enough oxygen to the cells, the respiration of the cells will be anaerobic respiration which produces lactic acid causing pain.

From that principle, oriental medicine has used many kinds of plants and grasses to make valuable medicines because they have medicinal properties that enhance blood circulation.

In addition to using plants and herbs as medicine, the Orient has practicing methods that with a Western perspective are mysterious, such as Yoga and Qi gong.

Yoga is a variety of movements and postures that essentially stretch muscles and joints, increasing blood circulation that carries nutrients and oxygen to the cells.

Qi gong also has many movements, in which the practice of breathing is the most important. Practice breathing is to breathe strongly and gradually air into the lungs, compressed it into the abdominal cavity for a while, then exhale gradually. According to physics, high pressure will increase the solubility of air in liquids. Thus, breathing practice also increases the flow of oxygen to the cells.

It is interesting because we see that Warburg's theory could also be the scientific basis for explaining the benefits of the above Yoga and

Qi gong practice. This is scientifically correct because when circulating blood does not bring enough oxygen to the cells, the cells will breathe anaerobically, a fermentation process that produces lactic acid causing pain and cancer.

As the introduction has written, practicing Yoga and Qi gong brings many health and spiritual benefits to the practitioner. Therefore, if we deeply understand the problem, we will know that breathing and exercising properly can also be a way to prevent and fight cancer. And as such, the air is the most valuable medicine and no payment to buy.

CHAPTER IV: THE EPIGENETIC CHANGES AND CANCER

1. What is epigenetic?

From the classical perspective, cancer is a collection of diseases caused by mutations of genes. Later, the role of epigenetic changes causing cancer was determined. Epigenetics are the study of phenotypic alterations that can be inherited without being involved in an alteration in the DNA sequence. These changes include DNA methylation and histone alterations that alter the activity of genes. These changes may remain when the cells are divided, exist for multiple pedigrees and can be considered to be epimutations (equivalent to mutations).

Cancer epigenetics is a field that studies the epigenetic alteration to the DNA of cancer cells. In a cell's transformation to cancer, epigenetic modification is important or even more important, than genetic mutations. Manipulation of epigenetic modification holds good promise for cancer preclusion, detection, and treatment.

Epigenetic aberrations modify DNA methylation, histone tails and regulate non-coding RNAs (microRNAs) - the parts that structure into chromosomes. Epigenetic changes occur a lot in the early stages of tumor formation and are an important factor in tumor growth. They can be reverted by "epigenetic drugs" because these drugs inhibit histone deacetylases and DNA methyltransferases.

Epigenetic drugs can restore genes, reverse the silence of tumor suppressors, help cells function normally back.

2. Structure of chromosomes

Each chromosome is constructed from two chromatids. The chromatid is made up of 60% histone proteins and 40% DNA.

DNA is a long polymer constructed from repeating units that are nucleotides. A nucleotide of DNA is made up of a phosphate group that links to the nucleoside formed from a sugar molecule that links to the nucleobase.

(Source: https://en.wikipedia.org/wiki/DNA#/media/File:DNA_chemical_structure.svg)

The polymer is called a polynucleotide that is the backbone of the DNA and contains nucleobases to interact with the nucleobases of the remaining DNA in the double helix through the hydrogen bonding system. Guanine pairs with cytosine and adenine pairs with thymine, denoted by G-C and A-T base pairs.

One DNA molecule coiled around eight histone molecules into nucleosome that is the basic unit of the chromosome.

The nucleosomes are joined together by DNA fragments and a histone protein to form a basic fiber with a width of 30 nm, which then twists three times to form a chromatid with a width of about 700 nm.

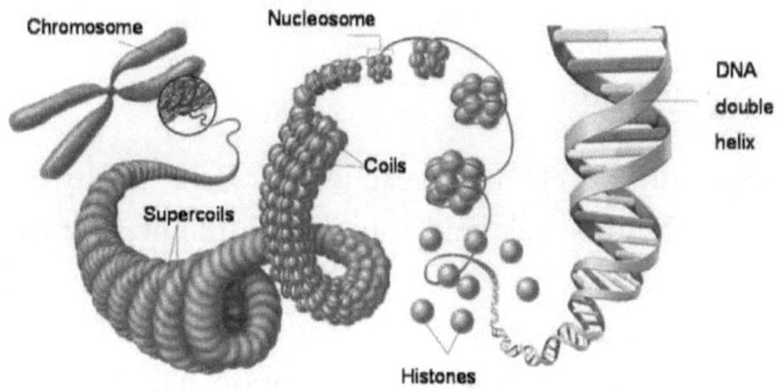

(Source: https://www.proprofs.com/discuss/q/690110/how-many-chromosomes-are-in-a-sperm-cell)

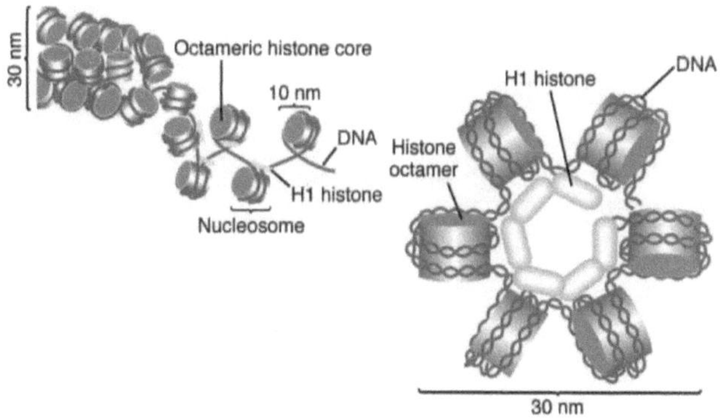

Source:

https://www.mun.ca/biology/scarr/Histone_Protein_Structure.html

3. The epigenetic mechanisms causes cancer

3.1. DNA methylation

DNA methylation is a chemical reaction in which methyl groups are inset to the DNA molecule and can change the activity of a DNA. Cytosine and adenine are two of DNA's four bases that can be methylated. DNA methylation attaches the methyl group to Cytosine in a gene promoter, repress gene transcription. DNA methylation is essential for normal action of DNA, but alterations of DNA methylation will cause cancer. That alterations are hypomethylation of oncogenes and hypermethylation of tumor suppressor genes.

The methylation process usually occurs at the 5 'position of cytosine in the CpG dinucleotides.

Cytosine   **methylated Cytosine**

"The CpG sites are regions of DNA where a cytosine nucleotide is followed by a guanine nucleotide in the linear sequence of bases along its 5' → 3' direction. CpG sites occur with high frequency in genomic regions called CpG islands (or CG islands). "

(Source: https://en.wikipedia.org/wiki/DNA_methylation)

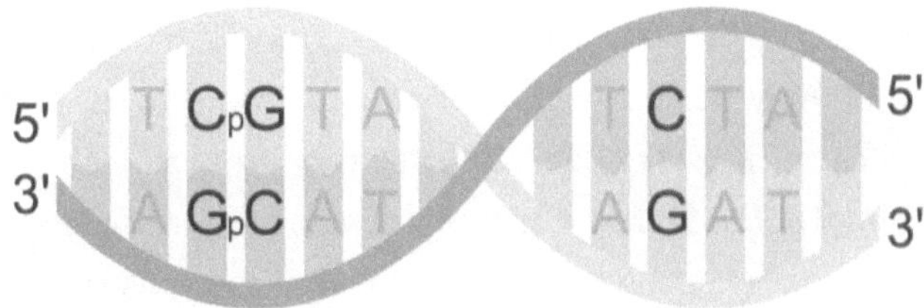

A CpG site, i.e., the " 5'—C—phosphate—G—3' " sequence of nucleotides, is indicated on one DNA strand (in yellow).

DNA methylation can result in the silencing of the genes. In normal cells, the methylation of CpG islands preceding gene promoters does not take place, but other individual CpG dinucleotides in the entire genome are methylated.

Methylation in cancer cells is just the opposite.

CpG islands preceding promoters of tumor suppressor gene are hypermethylated, can silence those genes, while CpG islands preceding promoters of oncogene are hypomethylated. These types of epigenetic changes cause cells to grow uncontrollably causing cancer.

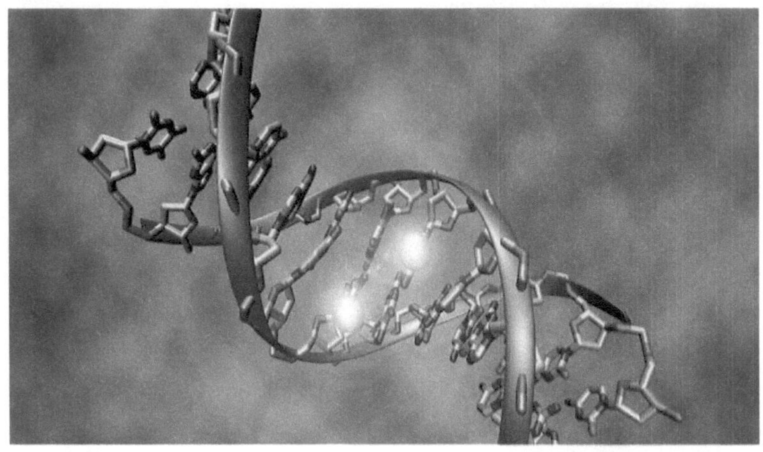

(Source: https://en.wikipedia.org/wiki/DNA_methylation)

DNA methylation was catalyzed by enzymes. It altered chromosome structure regulating gene expression patterns. Therefore, changes in the activity of enzymes can lead to the formation and development of various diseases. Throughout our life, the nutrients and biological substances in foods that affect enzymes can alter the global DNA methylation process involved in chromosome integrity and the causes of diseases.

3.1.1. The effect of nutrients on DNA methylation.

With the epigenetic field, enzymes that control the chemical reactions of epigenetic mechanisms can be directly affected by biologically active compounds, such as tea catechins and genistein that have an effect on DNA methyltransferase (Dnmt). Dnmts catalyzed the process of DNA methylation. Global DNA methylation can be altered throughout our lives by the foods we eat contain biologically active compounds that affect Dnmts. Global DNA methylation, which is related to the integrity of chromosomes as well as the DNA methylation of the gene-promoting region, is closely related to the activity of the oncogene.

Nutrients that contain folate, methionine, riboflavin, pyridoxine, cobalamin, choline, and betaine are components of the metabolism of a group of methyl. They are called "methyl donors".

S-adenosyl-L-methionine is a substance that is synthesized in the liver, providing methyl groups for methylation. In contrast, the active ingredients in the food also regulate levels of S-adenosyl-L-homocysteine, the enzyme inhibitor that catalyzes DNA methylation.

Folate is a water-soluble B vitamin, provides the methyl group to synthesize AdoMet, the only substance that provides methyl group for methylation reaction of DNA. Vitamin B-12, betaine, choline and methionine are also methyl donors that can change the process of DNA methylation.

Thus, theoretically, any nutrient, bioactive component, or condition that can affect AdoMet or AdoHcy levels in the tissue can alter the methylation of DNA.

Folate has an effect on the abnormal regulation of DNA methylation. The risk of a child having neural tube defects due to, in the early stages of pregnancy, the mother absorbs folate deficiency. Therefore, adding folate in the diet has been proposed to correct the errors of DNA methylation. The results of this study show that nutrients can alter the pattern of DNA methylation, which will have a positive effect on the development of a baby in utero and its health at birth and maturity. Spinach, lettuce, broccoli, orange, citrus, sunflower seeds, almonds, walnuts, macca, peanuts, citrus broccolirau spinach, salads, sunflower seeds, almonds, walnuts, macca, and peanuts are foods rich in folate.

Choline is a nutrient that provides the methyl group that a pregnant mother needs to be fully absorbed. It is essential for the development of the fetus's nerves as well as cognitive ability throughout life.

Soybean genistein, tea polyphenols or vegetable isothiocyanates can reduce the DNA hypermethylation in cancer-related genes, thus inhibiting the increase of cancer.

For instance, DNA methyltransferases are affected by tea catechin and genistein.

3.2. Modifying histone causes cancer

Modifying histone causes cancer The DNA of each of us can reach from the earth to the sun more than 600 times. Histone is what helps DNA fit into the nucleus of a cell.

Histones are proteins like a core (positively charged) and DNA like a thread (negatively charged), so histones bind with DNA very tightly like coiling the thread into chromosomes, squeezed into a tiny nucleus.

There is the only methylation in the DNA modification, while at the histon, its tail has different modifications such as acetylation, methylation, sumoylation, ubiquitination, biotinylation, phosphorylation and DP-ribosylation.

Abnormal modifications of histones will cause cancer. The active ingredients of food can also prevent those harms.

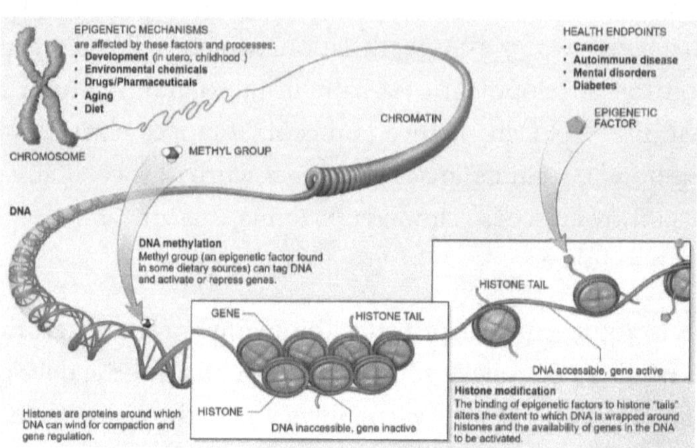

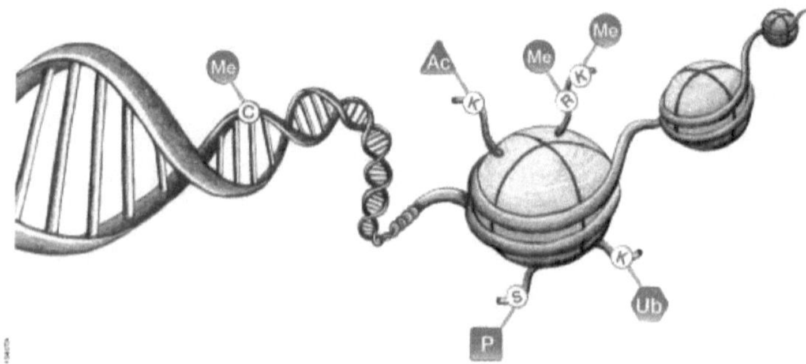

DNA methylation and histone modification: Me = methylation, Ub = ubiquitination, P = phosphorylation, Ac = acetylation.

(Source: https://www.promega.de/resources/guides/nucleic-acid-analysis/introduction-to-epigenetics/)

3.2.1. Histone acetylation and effects of nutrients

Cancer cells that regulate histone tend to differ from healthy cells.

Functional groups may be added or removed from the histone by several histone modification enzymes that affect the activity of genes wrapped around those histones.

Acetylation is the addition of the acetyl radical (-COCH3) to the tail of histone by the enzyme HAT (Histone Acetyltransferase). The acetyl group (-COCH3) is attached to the NH3+ position of lysine, neutralizes the positive charge, reduces the affinity between DNA and histone leads to loose DNA sequences (open chromosome, Euchromatin) which makes the genes are expressed. In contrast, deacetylation is the removal of acetyl radical (-COCH3) from the tail of histone by the enzyme HDAC (Histone deacetylase). This process makes the histone positively charged, increasing the affinity between DNA and histone resulting in tight DNA sequences (closed chromosome, heterochromatin) silencing genes that are not expressed.

Silencing the tumor suppressor genes and activating the oncogenes are the cause of cancer. Therefore, the researchers studied the activation of biologically active food ingredients on two enzymes HAT and HDAC because HDAC inhibition can "turn on" the silencing genes in cancer cells. Researchers have recognized HDAC inhibitors as substances that can cure cancer. Cancer cells grow and survive depending on HAT, so HAT also could be the target for drug development research to treat cancer.

Resveratrol, butyrate, sulforaphane, and diallyl sulfide can inhibit HDAC and curcumin can inhibit histone acetyltransferases (HAT). Altered enzyme activity by these compounds may affect physiologic and pathologic processes during our lifetime by altering gene expression. Turmeric contains curcumin, which has long been used as a medicine in Southeast Asia and India, as a HAT inhibitor.

Broccoli sprouts and broccoli contain sulforaphane, an isothiocyanate; Garlic contains an organosulfur, diallyl sulfide, and butyrate-containing fiber, an SCFA. Researched cell cultures have shown that sulforaphane downregulates deacetylation enzymes leading to inhibition of increase and growing of cancer cells. Vitamin D recruits histone acetylases. Other studies have studied the use of diallyl sulfide and butyrate to show a link between food and acetylation of histone. Grape skins contain resveratrol, a substance has anti-inflammatory and cancer effect because it inhibits inflammatory genes. Reprogramming in adult cells of humans may be caused by butyrate. Pantothenic acid is a fraction of CoA to create acetyl-CoA, which is a compound that provides an acetyl group for acetylation of histone. Water-soluble B vitamins like niacin, biotin, and pantothenic acid also can modify histone.

Enzymes associated with epigenetic mechanisms are affected by bioactive food ingredients. These compounds alter the enzyme activity that can affect physiological and pathological processes by altering gene expression.

3.2.2. Histone methylation and effects of nutrients

The change in histone methylation has been shown to have an effect on cancer and aging. The researchers studied the effects of nutrition on histone methylation.

S-adenosylmethionine (AdoMet) is a methyl donor for methylation reactions. If food is deficient in choline, a substance that supplies the methyl group, histone methylation will be reduced and affect fetal brain development. A diet that lacks methyl, folic, choline, and methionine, can cause liver cancer in research animals. This study demonstrates that histone methylation is affected by methyl deficient in the diet that causes the development of liver tumors.

Researchers also find a thing interesting that obesity is linked to histone methylation. In obesity and hyperlipidemia, the activity of metabolic genes is regulated by methylation status. The results of this study indicate that diets lacking methyl can affect methylation of histone causing liver tumors to develop. Also, there is a histone biotinylation. Biotin, a B vitamin, can change the tail of histones. Biotin deficiency in the diet can profoundly affect chromosome structure.

3.3. The abnormal regulation of MicroRNA causes cancer

3.3.1. What is MicroRNA?

MicroRNA is an unencoded small RNA molecule, approximately 21-25 nucleotides in length. These microRNAs control many different genes and many processes of the cell. If the miRNAs are altered, they will work more or less, which can affect the activity of their target genes and lead to various pathologies such as cancer, cardiovascular disease, and metabolic disorders. The activity of microRNAs can also be regulated by methylation of DNA or histone acetylation. Abnormal DNA methylation causes the epigenetic silence of miRNAs that frequently occur in cancer cells. DNA damage is the underlying cause of cancer. The altered expression of microRNA causes a deficiency of repair of damaged DNA that accumulates this damage which can also lead to cancer

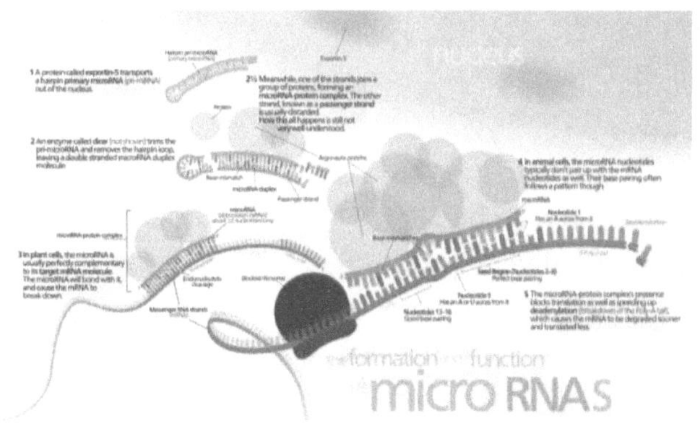

(Source: https://en.wikipedia.org/wiki/MicroRNA)

Depending on the effect of miRNAs, they may be considered as oncogenes or tumor suppressors. They are considered to be tumor suppressors if they slow down cell division or cause cell death.

Conversely, miRNAs are considered to be oncogenes if they increase cell division or cell survival. Many miRNAs activate so many different cancers. Some miRNAs that are epigenetically silenced early on in breast cancer may be as useful as tumor markers. MiRNA studies open up good prospects in many different areas of cancer diagnosis and treatment.

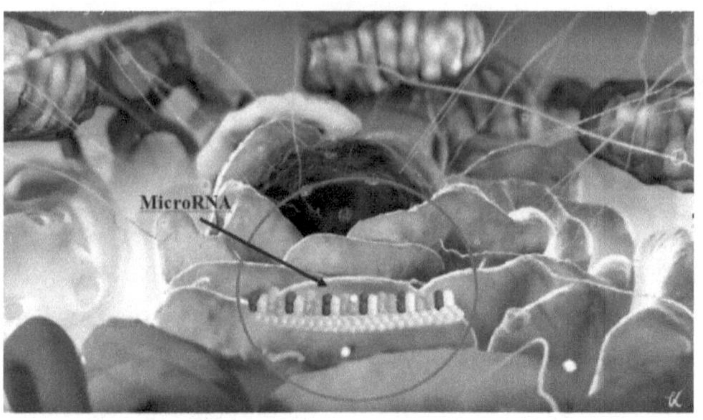

The activity of miRNA is influenced by our diet and therefore the risk of cancer can increase or decrease. Recent research results demonstrate that modulating miRNA expression by diet with sufficient nutrients such as curcumin, retinoids, and folate can be against cancer.

3.3.2. MiRNAs drive metabolism of tumor cell

For many years, researchers have known that cancer cells need more energy than normal cells (called the 'Warburg effect',) so cancer cells take up more sugar than normal cells. This energy is generated during the fermentation of sugar. The fermentation is an anaerobic process that produces lactic acid creating an acidic environment. Researchers have thought that miRNA causes the Warburg effect by affecting tumor suppressors such as p53.

3.3.3. MicroRNA as targets for cancer treatment

A large group of genes can be controlled by a single miRNA, so the drugs used to target miRNAs can be very effective.

Cancer treatment becomes difficult if the drug is resistant. Researchers have found that abnormal levels of many miRNAs promote drug resistance. However, when miRNA is restored to normal, it will increase the sensitivity of the drug back.

The modified level of non-coding RNA is controlled by various natural compounds.

Resveratrol regulates micro-RNA that affects the process that causes tumor growth or tumor suppression.

The altered expression of microRNA genes due to a diet lacking methyl (Nutrients containing folic acid, choline, and methionine, the "methyl donors") causes liver tumors in mice studied because it involves in regulating cell proliferation and apoptosis. These studies show that dietary methyl deficiency alters the activity of microRNA causing liver cancer and non-alcoholic steatohepatitis.

Some studies have suggested that the bioactive food ingredients (such as Genistein in soybeans, Curcumin in turmeric powder) that influence the activity of microRNAs may reduce the risk of cancer.

Folate in food regulates miRNA expression, which is effective in preventing cancer risk. In a folate-deficient environment, the level of miRNAs is altered, resulting in the development of human lymphoblastoid cells. If the diet is changed by the addition of folate, miRNA expression is reversible.

These results suggest that abnormal miRNA expression may be potential biomarkers leading to the use of nutritional status to prevent cancer. In HCC (hepatocellular carcinoma) there is a disruption of miRNA due to a diet lacking methyl (devoid of choline and folate and low methionine). When the mice with HCC were fed enough methyl, the activity of miR-122 (a miRNA) returned to normal and the tumors did not develop.

CHAPTER V: SOME FOODS THAT PREVENT AND FIGHT CANCER IN GENERAL

In order to use foods that effectively prevent and fight cancer during the meal, first of all, we need to avoid cancer-causing foods such as processed meats. The International Agency for Research on Cancer, under WHO, have classified them as Group 1 carcinogens such as ultraviolet light, cigarettes, and alcohol. (Cite: avoid-these-cancer-causing-foods). Processed meat is meat that has been smoked, salted, fermented, cured or improves preservation or enhances flavor, such as ham, sausages, lunch meats, and bacon. The risk of cancer in processed meats is due to the manufacturer adding nitrate preservatives to the meat. When we eat, nitrate changes into nitrite, which can increase the risk of cancer. Similarly, smoking bacon produces compounds that can cause cancer.

Researchers also advise us to eat less red meat and be careful when cooking them. Red meat is beef, pork, veal, lamb and goat. When these red meats are baked or cooked at high temperatures, they form heterocyclic amines and polycyclic aromatic hydrocarbons, which are carcinogenic compounds.

Researchers also advise us that should eat less sugar and the foods that can be converted into sugars such as starch.

According to Otto Warburg, cancer cells survive thanks to the fermentation of sugar. Some tests, which identify tumors on PET scans, have used radioactive glucose and found that cancer cells attract glucose faster than non-cancer cells. This process suggests cutting off sugar supply can starve and kill cancer cells.

In the body's metabolism, only carbohydrates are converted into sugar, so the proposed diet to fight cancer is to minimize carbohydrate intake and replace it with healthy fats like olive oil and avocados.

As the introduction has also written, there is no such kind of food as a miracle drug that can prevent and cure cancer. Regular use of a diet with just enough amount of meat and plenty of vegetables and tubers will be the best way for your body to be healthy and prevent cancer. This article will recommend top foods that can help us prevent cancer.

1. Mushrooms, tomatoes, carrots, red beetroot, broccoli, fatty fish, nuts, grapes, apple, blueberry, pomegranate, garlic, turmeric, ginger, green tea, supplements and medications

Mushrooms

are a food that has a delicate and unique flavor, so it has been a delicacy globally since ancient times. Recently, researchers have discovered that some mushrooms have anti-cancer effects.

Mushrooms contain active ingredients such as proteins, fats, polysaccharides, glycosides, alkaloids, phenolics, tocopherols, carotenoids, flavonoids, ascorbic acid, and enzymes. These ingredients have very valuable properties such as anti-oxidants, prebiotic, anti-inflammatory, anti-microbial, immunomodulating, anti-cardiovascular diseases, anti-diabetic and anti-cancer.

Tomatoes

Tomatoes are a commonly used vegetable that contains a lot of vitamin vitamins A, E and C, and carotenoids, including lycopene. Researchers have studied lycopene's anti-cancer properties.

Eating tomatoes has the strongest benefit for patients with prostate, stomach and lung cancer. One study found that tomatoes reduced the increase in liver cancer. Lycopene can make an important contribution to these benefits. But the researchers found that eating tomato powder was more effective than using the same dose of pure lycopene supplements. This proves that the other nutrients in tomatoes such as vitamins A, E, C, folate, phenolic compounds, minerals, and fiber also have anti-cancer effects, making the tomato anti-cancer effect stronger.

To maximize the benefits of lycopene and other carotenoids in tomatoes, oil-soluble substances, when cooking tomatoes, we should use a small amount of fat such as soybean oil, olive oil to dissolve them, and so they will be absorbed better when we eat.

Carrots

Carrots are a preferred vegetable that contains lots of Beta-carotene and alpha-carotene that our body converts into vitamin A, which is important for our body's function. It protects healthy cells by activating enzymes that are capable of metabolizing carcinogens.

Carrots also contain luteolin, a flavonoid compound that has antioxidant, anti-inflammatory and anti-cancer effects.

Researchers show that carrot carotenoids contribute to reducing cancer risk of oral, larynx, pharynx, and breast cancer. However, they recommend using foods rich in carotenoids because of their good synergistic effects, and should not use pure supplements such as beta-carotene when taken in high doses, which may increase the risk of lung cancer, especially is in smokers.

Carrots are a nutritious food, but they are low in calories, so adding carrots to our diet will keep us from becoming obese, which is the cause of many cancers.

Red beetroot

Red beetroot is a vegetable whose bioactive ingredients include carotenoids, saponins, polyphenols, flavonoids, saponins, and the main ingredient betaine.

Betaine is soluble in water and easily absorbed when we eat. Betalain has strong antioxidant properties, so it has a high ability to scavenge free radicals. In experiments, betaine reduced the DNA damage of liver cells during culture. It has been shown to induce detoxifying enzymes in cancerous liver cells, so it may have a protective effect on the liver and fight cancer in normal tissues.

Betaine also has strong anti-inflammatory properties. Researchers have found that betanin's anti-inflammatory ability is due to its strong removal of hypochlorous acid (HClO), a powerful oxidant produced by neutrophils.

Broccoli

In broccoli and cruciferous vegetables, there is a compound called sulforaphane that helps our body fight cancer. According to epigenetics, HDACs (Histone deacetylases) are enzymes that work against genes that prevent the increase of cancer tumors. The sulforaphane compound inhibits these HDAC enzymes.

Sulforaphane also has a property that normalizes DNA methylation, which abnormal DNA methylation will stimulate the onset of cancer. Therefore, sulforaphane prevents the activity of bad genes, helping cells to function normally.

Fatty fish

Fatty fish, including salmon, anchovies, and mackerel are rich in potassium, B vitamins, and especially omega-3 fatty acids.

The researchers found that people who ate a lot of fatty fish compared to those who ate less were less likely to suffer from cancers such as colorectal cancer, prostate cancer, and colon cancer.

Nuts

According to the researchers, all nuts have cancer-preventing properties, but walnuts are likely to be stronger than other nuts because they contain pedunculagin, a substance that can prevent breast cancer.

Legumes, such as peas, beans, and lentils, are high in fiber, which can help reduce the risk of developing cancers such as colorectal cancer and breast cancer.

Grapes

Grapes are not only a very delicious fruit, popular in the world, but also have great healing effects. Grapes contain resveratrol, a compound with powerful antioxidant and anti-inflammatory effects, and particularly its anti-cancer effects have been well studied. Researchers have shown that resveratrol can inhibit tumor formation of the liver, lymph, breast and stomach cells.

Scientists have also found that grapes contain other antioxidants in the flavonoid group. A team of researchers found that those chemicals work best together rather than as solitary substances. Grape extracts resist an enzyme that stimulates cell growth and reproduction. This enzyme is inhibited that can destroy cancer cells.

Apple

Apples contain Polyphenols that can prevent inflammation, cardiovascular disease, and infection, and especially against tumors. For example, a protein that helps cancer cells grow in some types of cancer called glucose transporter 2 (GLUT2) is inhibited by polyphenols.

The researchers also found in various antioxidants of apples there is a substance called Procyanidin, which is capable of activating a variety of cell signals that lead to the death of cancer cells.

Because of the valuable properties of apples, researchers claim that eating apples every day can reduce the risk of different types of cancer.

Blueberry

Blueberries contain antioxidants that provide countless health benefits. Recently, scientists have successfully extracted two important substances, Anthocyanin and Pterostilbene in Blueberry. They are used to produce drugs for the brain, neutralize free radicals, help limit vascular damage, protect and enhance brain activity. New studies have found that the active ingredients of Blueberries are also capable of treating cancer.

A research team tested blueberry extract on different types of human cancer cells. Separate blueberry extracts have helped reduce the number of cancer cells. When they used the blueberry extract in combination with radiation therapy, the results were better than taking them individually.

Pomegranate

Pomegranate contains powerful antioxidants such as anthocyanins, hydrolyzable tannins, and ellagitannins.

Studies have shown that pomegranate juice has anti-inflammatory effects and also has anti-cancer effects such as lung, prostate, breast, skin, and colon cancers.

Garlic

Global studies report that eating garlic regularly reduces the risk of colorectal cancer. Garlic compounds have been tested in the lab to show that they repair DNA, reduce inflammation and slow the increase of cancer cells.

Garlic compounds include S-allyl cysteine, allicin, flavonoids, inulin, and saponins. S-allyl cysteine is a water-soluble sulfur compound; while allicin is released when garlic is minced, forming some oil-soluble sulfur compounds that are the smell of garlic. Garlic flavonoids have two special substances, kaempferol, and quercetin, whose anti-cancer properties are well researched. Inulin is a carbohydrate that stimulates the increase of beneficial bacteria in the colon, which is good for health and prevents cancer.

In addition to reducing the risk of colorectal cancer, garlic is also being studied for its use in the prevention of other cancers.

Garlic is used primarily as the main spice in many Eastern dishes. It is used in cooking, pickled in vinegar or fermented into sour-flavored garlic to form a spice, used in meals.

Turmeric

Turmeric is a tuber that has been used as a spice in cooking and medicine for a very long time in Asian countries. Turmeric is used to treat arthritis, mixed with honey to cure stomach ulcers.

Today, modern science has identified turmeric containing the main active ingredient is curcumin. Curcumin is an antioxidant, has been shown to have anti-inflammatory properties and is especially able to prevent various forms of cancer. Curcumin has effects on various processes that are highly related to the growth and development of cancer cells, such as non-compliance with Apoptosis (programmed death), proliferation (an uncontrolled increase of cell), Angiogenesis (the process of creating lots of new blood vessels to nourish tumors) and chronic inflammation.

With such properties, Curcumin is good for prevention and fight against many different types of cancer, such as lung cancer, breast cancer, lymphoma and leukemia, melanoma, and ovarian cancer. and some other types.

"A Washington State University research team has developed a drug delivery system using curcumin, the main ingredient in the spice turmeric that successfully inhibits bone cancer cells while promoting the growth of healthy bone cells."

(Source: https://www.sciencedaily.com/releases/2019/06/190620121404.htm)

However, when they give patients oral curcumin as medicine, it was excreted too quickly. Therefore, 3D printing was used to create support frames from calcium phosphate combined with curcumin, contained in a bag of the fat compound into the frame, allowing gradual liberation of curcumin.

They found that the increase of osteosarcoma cells was inhibited by up to 96% after more than 10 days of treatment.

14. Ginger

Many health benefits of ginger have been recognized by different cultures through human experience from ancient times to the present day, but it was only recently that science been able to realize its anti-cancer properties. Even, according to a research result, the effect of ginger is 10,000 times stronger than that of a chemotherapy drug. (Cite: ginger-cancer-treatment)

Ginger contains 6-gingerol and 6-shogaol which have antioxidant and anti-cancer properties. A recent study indicated that 6-shogaol has powerful anti-cancer properties.

In addition to anti-cancer properties, Ginger also has antibacterial, antiviral, good for digestion, cardiovascular disease, asthma, enhances immunity and reduces pain.

Ginger is often used as a condiment to prepare the meat of some Eastern dishes. Ginger is also commonly used to make ginger jam candies and ginger tea. Drinking ginger tea is a great way to combat the onset of a cold and help reduce fever.

Green tea

In green tea, the main compound is (-) - epigallocatechin gallate (EGCG), which has been extensively studied by scientists around the world.

EGCG and green tea extract work to delay the onset of cancer, prevent the recurrence of colorectal adenoma, inhibit the spread of malignant tumor cells to the lungs, making increase the stiffness of lung cancer cells and inhibit their movement, and increase the effect when combining EGCG with other anti-cancer compounds.

Supplements and medications

Although we easily buy the foods, due to our lifestyles and taste, regular and adequate use of the foods listed above is not easy.

Those our shortcomings can be offset by the use of numerous supplements and drugs such as vitamins: C, A, E, and the plant-based compounds: anthocyanin, phloretin, and sulforaphane.

CONCLUSION

There is a paradox, the development of science and technology makes people's lives rich and comfortable, but it also creates many diseases of civilization such as obesity, diabetes, heart disease, and cancer. One of the main reasons is that people eat more and work less with muscles than when they are poor.

Many researchers believe that our modern food conflicts with ancient genes such as convenience foods and Fast Food. The American diet is filled with sugar and high energy drinks so many Americans are obese.

Researchers are becoming increasingly aware of how nutrition affects our genes. Nutrigenomics, a new field of science, was established to study the mechanism by which nutrition can protect genes from negative effects on genes due to lifestyle and the use of food containing toxic substances. Our genetic defects will be amplified increasing the risk of disease if we lack some essential nutrients.

This knowledge is really important because they enable us to design a diet and lifestyle strategy to help us fight diseases, including cancer.

Ho Chi Minh city, Viet Nam

February 12, 2020

DONG LA